Blue Collar Health

Blue Collar Health

Karen L. Aken

ISBN-13:978-1530267323
ISBN-10:1530267323

In loving memory of my Father,
Timothy R. Aken

Contents

Introduction

It has been estimated that 3.7 million people in America are living with an undiagnosed heart condition. I lost my Dad suddenly to undiagnosed heart disease in 2007. I always think about what he could have done differently to change the outcome. We thought he was healthy, unfortunately, he was under too much stress; never went to the doctor; and we missed several obvious signs. I became a health coach in 2015 so that I could prevent other people from experiencing a similar loss. I created this book with the hope that I could save or extend the life of at least one person who may also have undiagnosed heart disease or other disease brought on by an unhealthy lifestyle.

My Dad did not have type II diabetes, but I have included a bit of information about type II diabetes because it has become an epidemic in this country. According to the CDC, almost 10% of Americans have diabetes, and of that 10%, 30% don't even know they have it. I have kept the information that I feel everyone needs to know simple and straightforward. The information in this book can help prevent many diseases and lead to significant weight loss in individuals who are at an unhealthy weight. At the end of this book you will find 2 improved health/weight loss guides for people who cannot afford their own personal health coach, or simply want to improve their health on their own in the privacy of their own home.

The information in this book is not intended or implied to be a substitute for professional medical advice, diagnosis or treatment. All content contained in this book is for general information purposes only. Any reliance you place on such information is therefore strictly at your own risk.

1

Risk Factors for Heart Disease

- Stressful job or life
- Elevated LDL cholesterol
- High blood pressure
- Consistent lack of sleep
- Unhealthy sleep patterns
- Cigarette Smoking
- Lack of Physical inactivity
- Diet high in fat and/or high sodium
- Obesity
- Diabetes
- Family History
- Traumatic or unexpected loss of a loved one

Warning Signs of Heart Disease (please see a doctor if you have any of these symptoms)

- Chest pain
- Shortness of breath
- Pain, numbness, weakness, or coldness in legs or arms
- Pain in neck, jaw, throat, upper abdomen, or back
- Erectile dysfunction
- Lightheadedness, dizziness, fainting or near fainting
- Racing, slow, or irregular heartbeat
- Fluttering in your chest
- Swelling in your legs, ankles, and/or feet

- Blue or purple fingernails brought on by increased physical activity
- Fatigue
- Increased amount of belly fat (also referred to as a beer gut)
- Unusual amount of loss of fat or muscle on your hand in the area between your thumb and index finger. This was one of the few signs of heart disease my Dad had that I have never found in any textbook.

2

Risk Factors for Type II Diabetes

- Overweight or obese
- Unhealthy diet
- Lack of physical activity
- High blood pressure
- Family history
- Unhealthy sleep patterns
- Consistent lack of sleep
- Excessive alcohol intake

Warning Signs of Type II Diabetes (please see a doctor if you have any of these symptoms)

- Frequent urination
- Excessive thirst
- Increased hunger
- Weight loss
- Fatigue
- Tingling or numbness in hands or feet
- Blurred vision
- Slow-healing wounds
- Frequent infections
- Dizziness or ringing of the ears when you have waited to long to eat

3

How To Properly Check Your Blood Pressure

It is important to know what your blood pressure is because of the direct relationship between elevated blood pressure and heart disease. Blood pressure is generally recorded as two numbers, systolic blood pressure (SBP) and diastolic blood pressure (DBP). A check-up with your primary physician or other healthcare provider is best, but if you would like to keep track of your blood pressure with an at-home blood pressure monitor, please follow these steps:

1. Make sure the cuff size is appropriate for your arm. Arm circumferences of 22 to 26 cm need a cuff that is 12 x 22 cm (small adult); arm circumferences of 27 to 34 cm need a cuff that is 16 x 30 cm (adult); and arm circumferences of 35 to 44 cm need a cuff that is 16 x 36 cm (large adult) (Kaplan, 2010).
2. Sit with both feet flat on the floor for five minutes.
3. Smoothly and firmly wrap the blood pressure cuff around your arm with the lowest part of the cuff 1 inch above the inside of your elbow.
4. Make sure your arm is supported by an armchair or another person, keep your arm relaxed at an angle between 0 and 45 degrees and straight at the elbow.
5. Begin the blood pressure reading.

6. When complete, write down the numbers and then repeat steps on opposite arm. Contact your doctor if you have a difference of 15 mmHg or more between arms.

Adults 18 and over that have a systolic blood pressure less than 120 (mmHg) and a diastolic blood pressure less than 80 (mmHg) are classified as **Normal**.

Adults 18 and over that have systolic blood pressures between 120 and 139 (mmHg) and diastolic blood pressures between 80 and 89 (mmHg) are classified as having **Prehypertension**. People with prehypertension should schedule a checkup with their doctor.

Blood pressure readings for adults 18 and over that have systolic blood pressure between 140 to 159 (mmHg) and diastolic blood pressure between 90 and 99 (mmHg) are classified as having **Stage 1 Hypertension**. People with stage 1 hypertension should see their doctor immediately.

Blood pressure readings for adults 18 and over that have systolic blood pressure of 160 or above (mmHg) and diastolic blood pressure of 100 or above (mmHg) are classified as having **Stage 2 Hypertension**. People with stage 2 hypertension should see their doctor immediately.

Adults who have readings lower than the Normal classification should also check with their doctor to ensure their reading is not a cause for concern.

4

Stress Management

Stress management is one of the best ways to improve your overall health. I can always tell when someone is under a lot of stress because they usually have a belly that doesn't match the rest of their body. When people are under a great amount of stress, their cortisol levels rise, which leads to fat buildup around their midsection. Belly fat is dangerous because it surrounds your internal organs and suffocates them.

In order to reduce stress, your mind and body need downtime. When you set aside time to rest, your blood pressure will drop; your cortisol levels will drop; and your mind and body will relax and recoup. Five minutes of focused breathing in a quiet environment is more beneficial to your waistline than 500 sit-ups because it helps to lower cortisol and blood pressure. When you reduce cortisol levels, the fat that concentrates around your mid section (the stuff I like to call stress fat) will start to go away.

Focused breathing is simple. Shut off all devices (except for one that you will only use as a timer). Go somewhere quiet. Set your timer for at least 5 minutes. Sit comfortably. Close your eyes. Take deep breaths and focus only on the air coming into your nose, down into your lungs, and back out again. Try not to let your mind wander; be still and free of any thoughts. If your mind wanders, repeat a mantra until time is up. Use a mantra that is positive, if you prefer not to sound like a hippie by reciting "peace and love," recite things like "calm and patient," "free and clear," or "quiet and still."

Other ways to destress yourself are:

- Learn to say no to people who ask for more than you can give.
- Get a good night's sleep (see Chapter 5).
- Keep a note pad next to your bed. When problems or thoughts of what you need to get done pop into your head at night, write them down so that they can "get out of your head."
- Don't hold things in.
- Forgive others.
- When you are in a tense situation breathe slowly and deeply.
- Exchange time spent in front of the TV or online with time spent walking.
- Find creative ways to "kill two birds with one stone."
- Make a list of everything you do on a daily basis. Is there anything you can eliminate? Can you get help with anything on the list?
- Don't compare yourself or your life to others.
- Listen to music.
- Set aside time for a hobby that you enjoy.
- Don't dwell on the past.
- Limit social media.
- Talk about your problems to someone who will listen.
- Avoid people who stress you out.

- It's easier said than done, but if every single day you say you hate your job and you dread going to work, consider looking for a new one or switching to a different field. Workplace stress can lead to many health problems, including heart disease.

5

Get a Good Night's Sleep

No matter how busy your schedule is, you have to remember that sleep is just as important as a healthy diet or exercise. The following suggestions can help you achieve a better night's rest.

- Go to sleep at the same time every night and wake up at the same time every morning to keep your circadian rhythm (body clock) in check.
- Aim for 8 hours of uninterrupted sleep.
- Keep your room dark, turn any devices that emit light away from your eyes. Artificial light makes it hard for your brain to recognize that it is time for bed.
- Dim the lights and shut off electronic devices at least 30 minutes before bed.
- Turn down the thermostat, for optimal sleep keep the temperature in your bedroom around 66-67 degrees Fahrenheit.
- Avoid caffeine after 2 p.m.
- Keep your TV out of your bedroom.
- When you first lie down: breathe slowly for 5 seconds; hold for 2 seconds; and breathe out for 5 seconds. Repeat several times to relax your mind and body.

6

Exercise

The US Department of Health & Human Services recommends that adults engage in physical activity that adds up to:

- At least 2 hours and 30 minutes (per week) of moderate-intensity (ex. brisk walking); or 1 hour and 15 minutes (per week) of vigorous-intensity aerobic physical activity (ex. jogging); or an equivalent combination of moderate and vigorous intensity aerobic activity.

- For more extensive health benefits, adults should increase their aerobic physical activity to 5 hours (per week) of moderate intensity; or 2 hours and 30 minutes (per week) of vigorous intensity aerobic physical activity; or an equivalent combination of moderate and vigorous intensity activity.

- For additional health benefits, adults should also do muscle-strengthening activities that are moderate or high intensity and involve all major muscle groups on 2 or more days a week.

Avoid an all or nothing attitude. If you do not have enough time to exercise for an entire 30 - 45 minutes at one time, exercise in 10 minute bouts of moderate-intensity exercise throughout the day (i.e. brisk walk); or 7 minute bouts of vigorous-intensity exercise (i.e. up and down stairs).

Easy Ways To Increase Physical Activity

- At any time during the day do you wait for something? Maybe you are microwaving something. Whether it be for 30 seconds or 5 minutes, don't just stand there, march in place, do squats, or arm circles. Switch what you are doing for every 30 seconds you are waiting.
- Move things around your kitchen so that you have to walk back and forth. For example, if you make oatmeal every morning put your oatmeal in the left most cupboard, bowl in the right most cupboard, cinnamon back in the left, and so on. If you have a pantry, put items low so that you must do squats to get them. When you make your breakfast, grab each item one at a time.
- Keep a set of hand weights somewhere you know you will see them often. When you have a minute or two, do 10-12 repetitions of exercises such as bicep curls, tricep extensions, weighted squats, or shoulder presses.
- Park in the space farthest from the store, your workplace, and your front door.
- Always use the stairs instead of the elevator or escalator.
- Do side leg lifts or calf raises while brushing your teeth.
- Suck in your stomach off and on throughout the day for at least 30 seconds at a time. This will strengthen your stomach muscles and also improve your posture.
- Pay attention to how much time you spend on social media. Can you spend some or all of that time moving around instead?

- When you go to sit down, stand back up and sit down again a few times before you sit down for good. This will work your stomach, hips, thighs, and rear end. Do not do this exercise if you experience dizziness or nausea.
- Fidget more. Tap your toes, twist from side to side, chair dance, etc.
- Use the trip to the grocery store to add more steps to your day. Walk down every aisle.
- Bring in your groceries or other shopping bags one bag at a time.

8

Physical Activity and Working Full-Time

The demands of every occupation are different. If you have a physically demanding job, you need to rest more. If you have a mentally demanding job, but you are sitting all day, you need to move more.

Physically Demanding Job

- Stretch before, during, and after work.
- Breathe slowly and deeply on the drive into work.
- Use breaks to find "downtime" to sit and do breathing exercises in a quiet area or your personal vehicle.
- Massage sore legs, arms or feet during breaks using your hands, a rolled up towel, or a tennis ball.
- If possible bring a set of hand weights to work, during break, perform exercises that use muscles that are not used during a typical day of work to offset any muscular imbalances that have been created by overuse and repetitive motions.

Non-Physically Demanding Job

- Stretch before, during, and after work.
- Pay attention to your posture, sit straight, shoulders back.
- Stand at least once every half hour; every hour walk or march in place for at least one minute.

- Fidget as often as possible.
- Bring a portable lunch and walk during your break.
- Suck in your stomach and hold the position several times throughout the day.
- If possible bring a set of hand weights to the office. When you have a minute or two, do 10-16 repetitions of exercises such as bicep curls, tricep extensions, weighted squats, or shoulder presses.
- If you can't walk or bike to work because you live too far away, there is nothing saying you can't drive closer, park in a safe place, and finish your commute by walking or biking.

9

Water

I am a big fan of using water to improve your health. Depending on who you ask or what you Google, it is said that the human body is made up of about 60-75% water. So, it should only make sense that staying hydrated is one of the best things you can do for your body. Your body is an amazing machine. Every organ has a function and set of survival functions. Just like your car cannot run properly without oil, your body cannot run properly without water. **Men should drink at least 13 cups of water per day** and **women should drink at least 9**. The following are just some of the health benefits of staying well hydrated.

- Weight loss. Water helps you lose weight by keeping you feeling fuller longer.
- Lowers Blood Pressure. Our blood contains 92% water. Blood transports oxygen and nutrients throughout the body. When you are dehydrated your blood cannot transport the oxygen and nutrients your body needs as efficiently.
- Keeps you regular. Picture Play-Doh. When you were a kid if your Play-Doh was dried out could you squeeze it through any of those silly contraptions? When you don't drink enough water the colon pulls water from your stools to maintain fluids, essentially drying them out, just like Play-

Doh. If your stools are dried out, they won't be able to make it through any of your silly contraptions either.

- Reduces the risk of bladder and breast cancer. Water cleans out your system, the more you go, the faster you get rid of wastes and contamination.
- Improves mood. Dehydration can make you feel weak, tired, sick, and cause headaches. When you feel good your mood is good as well.
- Prevents headaches. When a piece of fruit is left out in the sun, the water leaves it, causing it to shrink and shrivel up. That's similar to what happens to your brain. Things tighten up when there is less water content, which causes things to ache.
- Keeps kidneys in check. Your kidneys are your body's filter. Drink plenty of water and your kidneys can do their job. Don't drink enough water and your kidneys have to work harder. They have to hold on to extra fluid so that they can perform their everyday functions. When you are well hydrated your urine will be light in color and odor free, dehydration will cause the opposite.
- Improves skin. Water reaches skin last. Staying well hydrated ensures that there is enough left over to provide hydration for your skin as well.
- Regulates body temperature. Your body needs water to sweat because sweat helps cool the body down.
- Lubricates joints. Your joints have a thin cushion of fluid to reduce friction during movement. That cushion is similar to a sponge, the less fluid you have, the smaller the sponge.
- Keeps us alert. Dehydration causes fatigue. Drink more water = feel less fatigued.

10

How To Read Nutrition Labels

I know that it is kind of a hassle to read nutrition labels, but if you typically buy the same products, you will only have to read the labels once. Here's an example of why it is important to read and understand nutrition labels:

A client once told me that he often ate a plate full of chicken nuggets for lunch because he considered chicken to be relatively healthy and he wanted the protein. He said he glanced at the nutrition label and thought chicken nuggets seemed ok. Let me just say that chicken nuggets are not in any way, shape or form a healthy option for a child or an adult. For every 5 nuggets there were 270 calories, 17 grams of fat, 4 grams of saturated fat, and 470 mg of sodium. He didn't think about the fact that he ate 12-15 chicken nuggets in one sitting, which meant that his lunch (on a day when he had 15 nuggets) contained 810 calories, 51 grams of fat, 18 grams of saturated fat, and 1,410 mg of sodium.

Nutrition Facts

Serving Size Do you actually eat the recommended serving? If the serving size says 1/4 cup and you are eating a full cup, get out your calculator and multiply the calories, total fat, cholesterol, sodium, carbohydrates, fiber, sugars, and protein by 4.

Carbohydrates Carbohydrates should make up 45-65% of your caloric intake. Carbohydrates provide 4 calories per gram, to determine your recommended intake take 45-65% of your total daily caloric intake and then divide that number by 4. If a product has a lot of carbohydrates and it's not a whole grain, potato, fruit or vegetable, try to avoid it.

Fat You need some fat in your diet, just make sure you are consuming "healthy" fats like monounsaturated and polyunsaturated fats found in things like nuts, seeds, avocados, and olive oil. Fat should make up 20-35% of your caloric intake. Fats provide 9 calories per gram, to determine your recommended intake take 20-35% of your total daily caloric intake and then divide that number by 9.

Saturated Fat Saturated fat raises blood cholesterol and your risk of heart disease. Choose products with less than 1 gram of saturated fat. One exception to the rule is peanut butter. Peanut butter will have slightly more than 1 gram of saturated fat.

Trans Fat Even worse than saturated fat, trans fat damages blood vessels, raises blood cholesterol, and raises your risk of heart disease. Choose products with 0 grams of trans fat.

Protein Protein should make up 15-35% of your caloric intake. Protein provides 4 calories per gram, to determine your recommended intake take 15-35% of your total daily caloric intake and then divide that number by 4. Intakes of 30-35% are only recommended for people who exercise for more than 60 minutes per day or who have a physically strenuous job.

Dietary Fiber The Institute of Medicine recommends that women aim to consume 25 grams of fiber per day, and men consume 38 grams per day. Fruits, vegetables, whole-grain foods, beans and peas are all good sources of fiber.

Cholesterol Similar to fat, cholesterol can also raise your risk of heart disease. You should aim to consume less than 300 mg of cholesterol per day.

Sodium High amounts of sodium raises blood pressure and puts a strain on your kidneys. Aim for less than 2,300 mg per day. For those with or at risk for heart disease keep sodium intake around 1,500 or less per day.

Sugar Avoid added sugars as much as possible. According to the American Heart Association, men should consume less than 37.5 grams or 9 teaspoons per day of sugar, and women should consume less than 25 grams or 6 teaspoons per day.

If you don't have time to read labels, the following are foods and drinks that have some of the highest amounts of sodium:

- Soup
- Cottage cheese
- Hot wings
- Fried Chicken
- Hot dogs
- Vegetable juice
- Sports drinks
- Frozen Dinners
- Chicken nuggets

- Deli meats
- Chicken pot pies
- Canned Vegetables
- Canned Tuna
- Pickles
- Olives
- Pretzels
- Salted Nuts
- Macaroni & Cheese

Most packaged foods and condiments have high amounts of sugar. The following are the foods, drinks, and condiments that have some of the highest.

- Yogurt
- Deli Meat
- Sports Drinks
- Milk
- Cereal
- White Bread
- Granola Bars
- Tomato Sauce
- Some Salad Dressings
- Ketchup

- Alcohol
- Canned Fruit
- Frozen Breakfast Foods
- Barbecue Sauce
- Instant Flavored Oatmeal
- Bottled Tea
- Soda
- Dried Fruit
- Energy Drinks
- Ice Cream

11

Breakfast

We have all heard it before, "Breakfast is the most important meal of the day." If you choose to make that breakfast a sugary cereal, it will quickly raise your blood sugar and give you an energy crash an hour or two later. Slow burning carbohydrates like oatmeal will prevent the quick rise in blood, prevent the energy crash, and help to keep you feeling fuller longer. If you truly prefer cereal, choose a fortified cereal that is low in sugar that can give you the majority of the nutrients you need. Just keep in mind that eating oatmeal every morning has been found to improve digestion, curb hunger cravings; and prevent heart disease, colon cancer and several other cancers.

A pooled analysis of cohort studies found that for every 10 gram increase of cereal fiber consumed per day, there is a 10% reduction in coronary heart disease events such as heart attack and stroke. (Pereira, 2004). The analysis also found that for every 10 gram increase of fruit fiber consumed per day, there is a 16% reduction in heart disease events (Pereira, 2004).

The following recipe is a great way to get both cereal fiber and fruit fiber:

- 1/4 - 1/2 cup gluten free quick oats
- 1/4 - 1/2 cup water
- 1/2 tsp cinnamon
- 1/2 cup frozen berries (strawberries are lowest in sugar)
- 1 tbs. peanut butter

Microwave for 2-3 minutes (all microwaves are different) stir in peanut butter after cooking.

12

Lunch

Keep it quick and healthy. A large lunch can make you feel lethargic and sleepy afterward. Frozen meals and fast food will contain high amounts of sugar and salt. Bring your lunch to work and choose healthier options such as the following:

The Main Course (choose one)

- Peanut butter on whole grain bread.
- 1 whole grain tortilla with 1/2 cup refried beans (choose vegetarian to reduce saturated fat) and 1/4 cup cheddar cheese. Throw in some peppers or onions if you can. Roll up or add another tortilla and make a quesadilla instead. Microwave for 30 seconds.
- Hearty salad. 1 to 2 cups red cabbage (cut in pieces or rip into smaller pieces with hands). 3 tbs. guacamole and/or 3 tbs. vegetarian refried beans. 1 tbs. salsa.
- Skip the BLT and go for a CLTC, cucumber, lettuce, tomato and cheese on whole grain bread.
- Tuna sandwich on whole grain bread (no pickles). Tuna has a high amount of sodium, but is ok to eat twice a week if you eat it on days when your sodium intake for other meals is low.
- Oatmeal Cookie oatmeal. 1/4 cup - 1/2 cup gluten free quick oats. 1/2 cup - 3/4 cup water. 1 tsp. cinnamon. 1/4 cup raisins or dried cranberries. 2 tbs. peanut butter. (this recipe has higher sugar content because of the dried fruit).

Sides (choose several, but only 1 type of nut)

- Baby Carrots
- Celery (can lower blood pressure)
- Radishes
- Cucumbers (can lower blood pressure)
- Whole Grain Crackers
- 24 Unsalted Almonds
- 14 Unsalted Shelled Walnut Halves (can improve sleep)
- 4 Unsalted Brazil Nuts (can lower cholesterol)
- 16 Unsalted Cashews
- 45 Pistachios
- Berries (low in sugar)
- Cantaloupe (low in sugar)
- Watermelon (low in sugar)

13

Dinner

A healthy meal is not one that is low in fat, carbs, and calories. A healthy meal is nutrient dense. When you fulfill your body's nutritional needs it can run more efficiently. You will find that you are less hungry; your metabolism will increase; and your immunity will improve.

To make the recipes you already have a bit healthier try some of the following ideas:

- Use ground turkey instead of ground beef
- Use Mrs. Dash instead of salt
- Buy organic
- Buy gluten free
- Use olive oil instead of canola or vegetable oil
- Bake instead of fry
- Cut out or cut back on the butter and salt
- Choose brown rice instead of white
- Always choose whole grain (look for the yellow whole grain stamp)
- Add frozen vegetables or frozen fruit whenever possible
- Avoid canned or if using canned rinse product to remove some of the sodium
- Use salsa or guacamole on salads instead of salad dressing

The following are just a few of my favorite nutrient dense recipes with simple ingredients that are easy to make.

White Chicken Chili (8+ servings)

- 2 cups vegetable broth
- 1 package McCormick White Chicken Chili Mix
- 1 lb. of diced or shredded chicken breast
- 2 - 15 oz cans great northern beans (drain and rinse well with water to eliminate most of the sodium)
- 1 - 15 oz can garbanzo beans (drain and rinse well with to eliminate most of the sodium)
- 1 can diced tomatoes and green chilies
- 1 - 8 oz bag frozen sliced mushrooms (optional)
- 1/2 cup diced onions
- 1/4 cup diced bell peppers (do not add until 20 min. before serving)
- 2 - 15 oz. cans of diced tomatoes (drained) or 2 cups of cherry tomatoes

Cook in a large crockpot on low heat for at least 5 hrs. stirring occasionally.

Thin Crust Pizza Burgers (5+ servings)

- 2 packages of Oroweat Multigrain Sandwich Thins
- Organic Pizza Sauce
- 1 Package of Shredded Mozzarella Cheese

Your choice of toppings: No canned veggies, instead choose tomatoes, frozen peppers, onions, and/or mushrooms.

Separate each sandwich thin into two halves, then add a spoonful of sauce, sprinkle on cheese, and add toppings. Bake for around 20 minutes at 400 degrees, because ovens vary check after 15 minutes.

Easy Bean and Chicken Enchiladas (5+ servings)

- 1 package whole grain tortillas
- 1 can of vegetarian refried beans (vegetarian means they were not cooked with animal fat)
- 1 package of Shredded Cheddar Cheese
- 1 lb. cooked chicken
- 1 bag of shredded carrots (optional)
- 1/2 cup diced onions (optional)
- 2 cans of enchilada sauce

Lay out tortillas. Spoon and spread refried beans onto each tortilla. Cover beans with a spoonful of enchilada sauce (use only 1 can, set aside other can). Cut up chicken into smaller pieces, evenly distribute over tortillas. Evenly sprinkle chopped onions over enchiladas (optional). Evenly sprinkle shredded carrots onto tortillas (optional). Evenly sprinkle cheese over tortillas, set aside small amount. Roll up tortillas and put into glass baking pan that has been sprayed with canola or olive oil no-stick cooking spray. Cover enchiladas with remaining can of sauce and sprinkle remaining cheese over the top. Bake at 400 degrees for 15 - 20 minutes.

Vegetarian Chili (8+ servings)

- 3 cans of chili beans (drained partially)
- 2 cans of black beans (drain and rinse to eliminate sodium)
- 1 bag of organic frozen corn
- 2 cans of diced tomatoes (drained) or 2 cups of cherry tomatoes
- 1/2 cup of diced onions
- 6 tbs chili powder
- 1 can tomato sauce
- 2 cans diced tomatoes & green chilies
- 1 cup sliced celery

Cook in crock pot over low heat for at least 5 hours stirring occasionally.

Simple Chicken (servings varied)

- 2 - 3.5 lbs uncooked organic chicken breasts
- 1 jar Salsa

Put chicken breasts in crock pot, coat with entire jar of salsa. Cook on low for 5 - 6 hrs.

14

Sunlight and Green Tea

Sunlight

Studies have correlated low vitamin D levels with a higher risk for cardiovascular disease. One of the easiest and cheapest ways to increase your vitamin D levels is to get it from sunlight. The "Health Professional Follow-Up Study" checked vitamin D blood levels in nearly 50,000 men who were healthy, and then followed them for 10 years (Giovannucci, 2008). They found that men who were deficient in vitamin D were twice as likely to have a heart attack as men with adequate levels of vitamin D (Giovannucci, 2008). So up your intake, five to fifteen minutes of sunlight on your arms, hands, and face two to three times per week is all you need.

Green Tea

Green Tea is a simple way to hydrate your body and reduce your risk for cardiovascular disease. A Japanese study found that those who consumed more than five cups of green tea a day had a 26% lower risk of death from a heart attack or stroke; and a 16% lower risk of death from all causes compared to people who drank less than one cup of green tea a day (Kuriyama, 2006). Green tea is most beneficial when served warm without extra flavoring. Bottled green tea will not produce the same benefits. If you find that you do not like the taste, be patient, within a week you will learn to tolerate if not enjoy the flavor.

15

Avoid Red Meat (or at least cut back)

To be honest, I hesitated putting anything about the avoidance of red meat in this book. I tell people to cut back on red meat and they stop listening to me, but the truth is, I wouldn't be able to live with myself if I didn't at least try to get the word out that red meat is just as bad, if not worse than smoking, stress, lack of physical activity, and fast food.

There are so many studies out there proving that red meat is bad for you that I could fill an entire book, but I won't. The study that stands out the most to me is one derived from two prospective cohort studies, The "Health Professionals Follow-Up Study" and the "Nurses' Health Study". Information from these two studies determined that people who ate the most red meat tended to die at a younger age, and died more often from cardiovascular disease and cancer (Pan, 2012). Their findings: each additional daily serving of red meat increased risk of death by 13%; the risk of death rose to 20% if the serving was processed, as in hot dogs, bacon, and cold cuts (Pan, 2012). Just to be clear, just ONE additional serving of red meat raised risk of death by 13% and just ONE additional serving of processed meat raised the risk of death by 20%.

Replace red meat with poultry that is not fried or breaded, oily fish that is baked or steamed instead of fried (2x per week), or beans and brown rice.

16

Start Your Journey To Improved Health

Prepare your own schedule, setting aside time for increased physical activity, downtime, and healthy eating habits or follow one of my improved health/weight loss guides.

Before You Start
- Check with your doctor before beginning these or any other exercise programs.
- Understand that rapid weight loss of more than 1.5 to 2 lbs. per week or weight loss of more than 1% of your body weight may cause serious health problems.
- Remember to breathe when lifting weights, never hold your breath, strain, or grip the weights too tightly.
- Know that only permanent lifestyle changes: making healthy food choices and increasing physical activity promote long term weight loss.
- If you feel dizzy, short of breath, or experience nausea at any time during physical activity stop immediately. If these symptoms are accompanied by chest pain or tightness go to the emergency room or call emergency medical help right away.
- Always warmup before a workout and cool down after.
- When lifting weights: once repetitions become too easy (you can do more than 20 reps easily), increase the weight.
- The information in this book is not intended or implied to be a substitute for professional medical advice, diagnosis

or treatment. All content contained in this book is for general information purposes only. Any reliance you place on such information is therefore strictly at your own risk.

17

Beginner Improved Health/Weight Loss Program

This program is meant only for individuals that do not currently engage in physical activity and do not consume a healthy diet on a regular basis. This program is not intended to create rapid weight loss, it is intended to improve your health significantly and create a slow, healthy weight loss that can be maintained for the rest of your life. You may or may not see any weight loss within the first 2 weeks, but you will feel a difference in your energy and your mood. When you do begin to lose weight, please keep in mind that a healthy weight loss is only about 1.5 to 2 lbs. per week. Losing weight slowly will increase your chances that it will stay off. Check with your doctor before beginning this or any other exercise program.

Week 1

- Walk for 10 minutes every day.
- Females drink 7 cups of water and 1 cup of green tea every day. Males drink 9 cups of water and 1 cup of green tea every day.
- Set aside 5 minutes every day for focused breathing. Shut off all devices (except for one that you will only use as a timer). Go somewhere quiet. Set your timer. Sit comfortably. Close your eyes. Take deep breaths and focus only on the air coming into your nose, down into your lungs, and back out again. Try not to let your mind wander; be still and free of any thoughts. If you need to quiet your mind, repeat your own mantra if needed.
- Find 5 minutes every day to spend in the sun.
- Change one meal, try eating oatmeal for breakfast or lunch. Your willpower will be strongest in the morning.
- Make sure you are eating at least one fruit and one vegetable every day.

Week 2

- Eat oatmeal for breakfast every day.
- Walk for 10 minutes every day.
- Get a set of hand weights that you can lift comfortably, but still give you a slight challenge. Perform 1 set (12-15 reps) of bicep curls. Perform this exercise every day or every other day.
- Females drink 7 cups of water and 2 cups of green tea every day. Males drink 9 cups of water and 2 cups of green tea every day.
- Set aside 5 minutes every day for focused breathing.
- Find 5 minutes every day to spend in the sun.
- If you typically eat red meat every day, aim to cut out red meat for an entire day at least once this week.
- Make sure you are eating at least one fruit and one vegetable every day.

Week 3

- Eat oatmeal for breakfast every day.
- Walk for 15 minutes every day.
- Perform 1 set (12-15 reps) of bicep curls. Perform this exercise every day or every other day.
- Females drink 6 cups of water and 3 cups of green tea every day. Males drink 9 cups of water and 3 cups of green tea every day.
- Set aside 5 minutes every day for focused breathing.
- Find 5 minutes every day to spend in the sun.
- If you typically eat red meat every day, aim to cut out red meat for an entire day at least once this week.
- Make sure you are eating at least one fruit and two different types of vegetables every day.

Week 4

- Eat oatmeal for breakfast every day.
- Walk for 15 minutes every day.
- Perform 2 sets (12-15 reps) of bicep curls. Perform 1 set of tricep kickbacks (10-12 reps). Perform these exercises every other day. Rest for at least 60 seconds between sets.
- Females drink 6 cups of water and 3 cups of green tea every day. Males drink 10 cups of water and 3 cups of green tea every day.
- Set aside 5 minutes every day for focused breathing.
- Find 5 minutes every day to spend in the sun.
- If you typically eat red meat every day, aim to cut out red meat for an entire day at least 2x this week.
- Make sure you are eating at least one fruit and two different types of vegetables every day.

Week 5

- Eat oatmeal for breakfast every day.
- Walk for 20 minutes every day (can be split into 2 - 10 minute sessions).
- Perform 2 sets (12-15 reps) of bicep curls. Perform 1 set of tricep kickbacks (10-12 reps). Perform these exercises every other day. Rest for at least 60 seconds between sets.
- Females drink 6 cups of water and 3 cups of green tea every day. Males drink 10 cups of water and 3 cups of green tea every day.
- Set aside 5 minutes every day for focused breathing.
- Find 5 minutes every day to spend in the sun.
- If you typically eat red meat every day, aim to cut out red meat for an entire day at least 2x this week.
- Make sure you are eating at least two different fruits and two different types of vegetables every day.

Week 6

- Eat oatmeal for breakfast every day.
- Walk for 20 minutes every day (can be split into 2 - 10 minute sessions).
- Perform 3 sets (12-15 reps) of bicep curls. Perform 2 sets of tricep kickbacks (10-12 reps). Perform these exercises every other day. Rest for at least 60 seconds between sets.
- Females drink 6 cups of water and 3 cups of green tea every day. Males drink 10 cups of water and 3 cups of green tea every day.
- Set aside 5 minutes every day for focused breathing.
- Find 5 minutes every day to spend in the sun.
- If you typically eat red meat every day, aim to cut out red meat for an entire day at least 3x this week.
- Make sure you are eating at least two different fruits and two different types of vegetables every day.

Week 7

- Eat oatmeal for breakfast every day.
- Walk for 25 minutes every day (can be split into 2 - 10 minute sessions).
- Perform 3 sets (12-15 reps) of bicep curls. Perform 2 sets of tricep kickbacks (10-12 reps). Perform these exercises every other day. Rest for at least 60 seconds between sets.
- Females drink 6 cups of water and 3 cups of green tea every day. Males drink 10 cups of water and 3 cups of green tea every day.
- Set aside 6 minutes every day for focused breathing.
- Find 5 minutes every day to spend in the sun.
- If you typically eat red meat every day, aim to cut out red meat for an entire day at least 3x this week.
- Make sure you are eating at least two different fruits and three different types of vegetables every day.

Week 8

- Eat oatmeal for breakfast every day.
- Walk for 25 minutes every day (can be split into 2 - 10 minute sessions).
- Perform 3 sets (12-15 reps) of bicep curls. Perform 3 sets of tricep kickbacks (10-12 reps). Perform 1 set of overhead presses (12-15 reps). Perform these exercises every other day. Rest for at least 60 seconds between sets.
- Females drink 6 cups of water and 3 cups of green tea every day. Males drink 10 cups of water and 3 cups of green tea every day.
- Set aside 6 minutes during every day for focused breathing.
- Find 5 minutes every day to spend in the sun.
- If you typically eat red meat every day, aim to cut out red meat for an entire day at least 4x this week.
- Make sure you are eating at least two different fruits and three different types of vegetables every day.

Week 9

- Eat oatmeal for breakfast every day.
- Walk for 30 minutes every day (can be split into 2 sessions).
- Perform 3 sets (12-16 reps) of bicep curls. Perform 3 sets of tricep kickbacks (10-12 reps). Perform 1 set of overhead presses (10-12 reps). Perform these exercises every other day. Rest for at least 60 seconds between sets.
- Females drink 6 cups of water and 3 cups of green tea every day. Males drink 10 cups of water and 3 cups of green tea every day.
- Set aside 6 minutes every day for focused breathing.
- Find 5 minutes every day to spend in the sun.
- If you typically eat red meat every day, aim to cut out red meat for an entire day at least 4x this week.
- Make sure you are eating at least three servings of fruit and three servings of vegetables every day. 1 serving of fruit = 1 cup, 1 serving of vegetables = 1/2 cup.

Week 10

- Eat oatmeal for breakfast every day.
- Walk for 30 minutes every day (can be split into 2 sessions).
- Perform 3 sets (12-16 reps) of bicep curls. Perform 3 sets of tricep kickbacks (10-12 reps). Perform 2 sets of overhead presses (10-12 reps). Perform these exercises every other day. Rest for at least 60 seconds between sets.
- Females drink 6 cups of water and 3 cups of green tea every day. Males drink 10 cups of water and 3 cups of green tea every day.
- Set aside 6 minutes every day for focused breathing.
- Find 5 minutes every day to spend in the sun.
- If you typically eat red meat every day, aim to cut out red meat for an entire day at least 5x this week.
- Make sure you are eating at least three servings of fruit and three servings of vegetables every day. 1 serving of fruit = 1 cup, 1 serving of vegetables = 1/2 cup.

Week 11

- Eat oatmeal for breakfast every day.
- Walk for 35 minutes every day (can be split into 2 sessions).
- Perform 3 sets (12-16 reps) of bicep curls. Perform 3 sets of tricep kickbacks (10-12 reps). Perform 2 sets of overhead presses (10-12 reps). Perform these exercises every other day. Rest for at least 60 seconds between sets.
- Females drink 6 cups of water and 3 cups of green tea every day. Males drink 10 cups of water and 3 cups of green tea every day.
- Set aside 6 minutes every day for focused breathing.
- Find 5 minutes every day to spend in the sun.
- If you typically eat red meat every day, aim to cut out red meat for an entire day at least 5x this week.
- Make sure you are eating at least three servings of fruit and three servings of vegetables every day. 1 serving of fruit = 1 cup, 1 serving of vegetables = 1/2 cup.

Week 12

- Eat oatmeal for breakfast every day.
- Walk for 35 minutes every day (can be split into 2 sessions).
- Perform 3 sets (12-16 reps) of bicep curls. Perform 3 sets of tricep kickbacks (12-16 reps). Perform 2 sets of overhead presses (10-12 reps). Perform these exercises every other day. Rest for at least 60 seconds between sets.
- Females drink 6 cups of water and 3 cups of green tea every day. Males drink 10 cups of water and 3 cups of green tea every day.
- Set aside 6 minutes every day for focused breathing.
- Find 5 minutes every day to spend in the sun.
- If you typically eat red meat every day, aim to cut out red meat for an entire day at least 5x this week.
- Make sure you are eating at least three servings of fruit and four servings of vegetables every day. 1 serving of fruit = 1 cup, 1 serving of vegetables = 1/2 cup.

Week 13

- Eat oatmeal for breakfast every day.
- Walk for 40 minutes every day (can be split into 2 sessions).
- Perform 3 sets (12-16 reps) of bicep curls. Perform 3 sets of tricep kickbacks (12-16 reps). Perform 3 sets of overhead presses (10-12 reps). Perform these exercises every other day. Rest for at least 60 seconds between sets.
- Perform 1 set of bodyweight squats (10-12 reps) every day. Keep your back straight, your spine neutral, and your chest and shoulders up. Look straight ahead throughout squat. As you squat down, focus on keeping your knees in line with your feet.
- Females drink 6 cups of water and 3 cups of green tea every day. Males drink 10 cups of water and 3 cups of green tea every day.
- Set aside 7 minutes every day for focused breathing.
- Find 5 minutes every day to spend in the sun.
- If you typically eat red meat every day, aim to cut out red meat for an entire day at least 5x this week.
- Make sure you are eating at least three servings of fruit and four servings of vegetables every day. 1 serving of fruit = 1 cup, 1 serving of vegetables = 1/2 cup.

Week 14

- Eat oatmeal for breakfast every day.
- Walk for 40 minutes every day (can be split into 2 sessions).
- Perform 3 sets (12-16 reps) of bicep curls. Perform 3 sets of tricep kickbacks (12-16 reps). Perform 3 sets of overhead presses (10-12 reps). Perform these exercises every other day. Rest for at least 60 seconds between sets.
- Perform 1 set of bodyweight squats (10-12 reps) every day.
- Females drink 6 cups of water and 3 cups of green tea every day. Males drink 10 cups of water and 3 cups of green tea every day.
- Set aside 7 minutes every day for focused breathing.
- Find 5 minutes every day to spend in the sun.
- If you typically eat red meat every day, aim to cut out red meat for an entire day at least 5x this week.
- Make sure you are eating at least three servings of fruit and four servings of vegetables every day. 1 serving of fruit = 1 cup, 1 serving of vegetables = 1/2 cup.

Week 15

- Eat oatmeal for breakfast every day.
- Walk for 45 minutes every day (can be split into 2 sessions).
- Perform 3 sets (12-16 reps) of bicep curls. Perform 3 sets of tricep kickbacks (12-16 reps). Perform 3 sets of overhead presses (12-16 reps). Perform these exercises every other day. Rest for at least 60 seconds between sets.
- Perform 2 sets of bodyweight squats (10-12 reps) every day.
- Females drink 6 cups of water and 3 cups of green tea every day. Males drink 10 cups of water and 3 cups of green tea every day.
- Set aside 7 minutes every day for focused breathing.
- Find 5 minutes every day to spend in the sun.
- If you typically eat red meat every day, aim to cut out red meat for an entire day at least 5x this week.
- Make sure you are eating at least three servings of fruit and four servings of vegetables every day. 1 serving of fruit = 1 cup, 1 serving of vegetables = 1/2 cup.

Week 16

- Eat oatmeal for breakfast every day.
- Walk for 45 minutes every day (can be split into 2 sessions).
- Perform 3 sets (12-16 reps) of bicep curls. Perform 3 sets of tricep kickbacks (12-16 reps). Perform 3 sets of overhead presses (12-16 reps). Perform these exercises every other day. Rest for at least 60 seconds between sets.
- Perform 2 sets of bodyweight squats (10-12 reps) every day.
- Females drink 6 cups of water and 3 cups of green tea every day. Males drink 10 cups of water and 3 cups of green tea every day.
- Set aside 7 minutes every day for focused breathing.
- Find 5 minutes every day to spend in the sun.
- If you typically eat red meat every day, aim to cut out red meat for an entire day at least 5x this week.
- Make sure you are eating at least three servings of fruit and four servings of vegetables every day. 1 serving of fruit = 1 cup, 1 serving of vegetables = 1/2 cup.

Week 17

- Eat oatmeal for breakfast every day.
- Walk for 45 minutes every day (can be split into 2 sessions).
- Perform 3 sets (12-16 reps) of bicep curls. Perform 3 sets of tricep kickbacks (12-16 reps). Perform 3 sets of overhead presses (12-16 reps). Perform these exercises every other day. Rest for at least 60 seconds between sets.
- Perform 3 sets of bodyweight squats (10-12 reps) every day.
- Females drink 6 cups of water and 3 cups of green tea every day. Males drink 10 cups of water and 3 cups of green tea every day.
- Set aside 7 minutes every day for focused breathing.
- Find 5 minutes every day to spend in the sun.
- If you typically eat red meat every day, aim to cut out red meat for an entire day at least 5x this week.
- Make sure you are eating at least three servings of fruit and four servings of vegetables every day. 1 serving of fruit = 1 cup, 1 serving of vegetables = 1/2 cup.

Week 18

- Eat oatmeal for breakfast every day.
- Walk for 45 minutes every day (can be split into 2 sessions).
- Perform 3 sets (12-16 reps) of bicep curls. Perform 3 sets of tricep kickbacks (12-16 reps). Perform 3 sets of overhead presses (12-16 reps). Perform these exercises every other day. Rest for at least 60 seconds between sets.
- Perform 3 sets of bodyweight squats (10-12 reps) every day.
- Females drink 6 cups of water and 3 cups of green tea every day. Males drink 10 cups of water and 3 cups of green tea every day.
- Set aside 7 minutes every day for focused breathing.
- Find 5 minutes every day to spend in the sun.
- If you typically eat red meat every day, aim to cut out red meat for an entire day at least 5x this week.
- Make sure you are eating at least three servings of fruit and four servings of vegetables every day. 1 serving of fruit = 1 cup, 1 serving of vegetables = 1/2 cup.

Week 19

- Eat oatmeal for breakfast every day.
- Walk for 45 minutes every day (can be split into 2 sessions).
- Perform 3 sets (12-16 reps) of bicep curls. Perform 3 sets of tricep kickbacks (12-16 reps). Perform 3 sets of overhead presses (12-16 reps). Perform these exercises every other day. Rest for at least 60 seconds between sets.
- Perform 3 sets of bodyweight squats (12-16 reps) every day.
- Females drink 6 cups of water and 3 cups of green tea every day. Males drink 10 cups of water and 3 cups of green tea every day.
- Set aside 7 minutes every day for focused breathing.
- Find 5 minutes every day to spend in the sun.
- If you typically eat red meat every day, aim to cut out red meat for an entire day at least 5x this week.
- Make sure you are eating at least three servings of fruit and four servings of vegetables every day. 1 serving of fruit = 1 cup, 1 serving of vegetables = 1/2 cup.

Week 20

- Eat oatmeal for breakfast every day.
- Walk for 45 minutes every day (can be split into 2 sessions).
- Perform 3 sets (12-16 reps) of bicep curls. Perform 3 sets of tricep kickbacks (12-16 reps). Perform 3 sets of overhead presses (12-16 reps). Perform these exercises every other day. Rest for at least 60 seconds between sets.
- Perform 3 sets of bodyweight squats (12-16 reps) every day.
- Females drink 6 cups of water and at least 3 cups of green tea every day. Males drink 10 cups of water and at least 3 cups of green tea every day.
- Set aside 7 minutes every day for focused breathing.
- Find 5 minutes every day to spend in the sun.
- If you typically eat red meat every day, aim to cut out red meat for an entire day at least 5x per week.
- Make sure you are eating at least three servings of fruit and four servings of vegetables every day. 1 serving of fruit = 1 cup, 1 serving of vegetables = 1/2 cup.

From now on: continue with Week 20, adjusting the amount of weight, sets, or repetitions as needed; or create your own program based upon your abilities, likes, and dislikes.

18

Advanced Improved Health/Weight Loss Program

This program is meant only for individuals that have no trouble walking briskly for 20 minutes, but do not consume a healthy diet on a regular basis. This program is not for individuals with uncontrolled diabetes or heart disease. This program is not intended to create rapid weight loss, it is intended to improve your health significantly and create a slow, healthy weight loss that can be maintained for the rest of your life. You may or may not see any weight loss within the first 2 weeks, but you will feel a difference in your energy and your mood. When you do begin to lose weight, please keep in mind that a healthy weight loss is only about 1.5 to 2 lbs. per week. Losing weight slowly increases your chances that it will stay off. Check with your doctor before beginning this or any other exercise program.

Week 1

- Walk briskly for 20 minutes every day.
- Females drink 6 cups of water and 2 cups of green tea every day. Males drink 10 cups of water and 2 cups of green tea every day.
- Set aside 5 minutes for focused breathing every day. Shut off all devices (except one that you will only use as a timer). Go somewhere quiet. Set your timer. Sit comfortably. Close your eyes. Take deep breaths and focus only on the air coming into your nose, down into your lungs, and back out again. Try not to let your mind wander; be still and free of any thoughts. If you need to quiet your mind, repeat your own mantra if needed.
- Get a set of hand weights that you can lift comfortably, but still give you a slight challenge. If you can lift them with more than 20x with ease, they are too light. Perform 1 set (12-16 reps) of bicep curls. Perform 1 set of overhead presses (12-16 reps). Perform 1 set (10-16 reps) of tricep kickbacks or overhead tricep extensions. Perform these exercises every other day.
- Find 5 minutes every day to spend in the sun.
- Change one meal, try eating oatmeal for breakfast or lunch. Your willpower will be strongest in the morning.
- If you typically eat red meat every day, aim to cut out red meat for an entire day at least once this week.
- Make sure you are eating at least one serving of fruit and one serving of vegetables every day.

Week 2

- Eat oatmeal for breakfast every day.
- Walk briskly for 20 minutes every day.
- Get a set of hand weights that you can lift comfortably, but gives you a slight challenge. Perform 1 set (12-16 reps) of bicep curls. Perform 1 set of overhead presses (12-16 reps). Perform 1 set (10-16 reps) of tricep kickbacks or overhead tricep extensions. Perform these exercises every other day.
- Perform 1 set of bodyweight squats (10-12 reps) every day. Keep your back straight, your spine neutral, and your chest and shoulders up. Look straight ahead throughout squat. As you squat down, focus on keeping your knees in line with your feet.
- Females drink 6 cups of water and 2 cups of green tea every day. Males drink 10 cups of water and 2 cups of green tea every day.
- Set aside 5 minutes every day for focused breathing.
- Find 5 minutes every day to spend in the sun.
- If you typically eat red meat every day, aim to cut out red meat for an entire day at least once this week.
- Make sure you are eating at least one serving of fruit and one serving of vegetables every day.

Week 3

- Eat oatmeal for breakfast every day.
- Walk briskly for 20 minutes every day.
- Perform 1 set (12-16 reps) of bicep curls. Perform 1 set of overhead presses (12-16 reps). Perform 1 set (10-16 reps) of tricep kickbacks or overhead tricep extensions. Perform these exercises every other day.
- Perform 1 set of bodyweight squats (12-15 reps) every day.
- Females drink 6 cups of water and 3 cups of green tea every day. Males drink 10 cups of water and 3 cups of green tea every day.
- Set aside 5 minutes every day for focused breathing.
- Find 5 minutes every day to spend in the sun.
- If you typically eat red meat every day, aim to cut out red meat for an entire day at least 2x this week.
- Make sure you are eating at least one serving of fruit and two servings of vegetables every day.

Week 4

- Eat oatmeal for breakfast every day.
- Walk briskly for 25 minutes every day.
- Perform 2 sets (12-16 reps) of bicep curls. Perform 2 sets of overhead presses (12-16 reps). Perform 2 sets (10-16 reps) of tricep kickbacks or overhead tricep extensions. Perform these exercises every other day. Rest for at least 60 seconds between sets.
- Perform 1 set of bodyweight squats (10-12 reps) every day.
- Females drink 6 cups of water and 3 cups of green tea every day. Males drink 10 cups of water and 3 cups of green tea every day.
- Set aside 5 minutes every day for focused breathing.
- Find 5 minutes every day to spend in the sun.
- If you typically eat red meat every day, aim to cut out red meat for an entire day at least 2x this week.
- Make sure you are eating at least one serving of fruit and two servings of vegetables every day.

Week 5

- Eat oatmeal for breakfast every day.
- Walk briskly for 25 minutes every day.
- Perform 2 sets (12-16 reps) of bicep curls. Perform 2 sets of overhead presses (12-16 reps). Perform 2 sets (10-16 reps) of tricep kickbacks or overhead tricep extensions. Perform these exercises every other day. Rest for at least 60 seconds between sets.
- Perform 2 sets of bodyweight squats (10-12 reps) every day. Rest for at least 60 seconds between sets.
- Females drink 6 cups of water and 3 cups of green tea per day. Males drink 10 cups of water and 3 cups of green tea per day.
- Set aside 5 minutes every day for focused breathing.
- Find 5 minutes every day to spend in the sun.
- If you typically eat red meat every day, aim to cut out red meat for an entire day at least 3x this week.
- Make sure you are eating at least two servings of fruit and two servings of vegetables every day.

Week 6

- Eat oatmeal for breakfast every day.
- Walk briskly for 25 minutes every day.
- Perform 3 sets (12-16 reps) of bicep curls. Perform 3 sets of overhead presses (12-16 reps). Perform 3 sets (10-16 reps) of tricep kickbacks or overhead tricep extensions. Perform these exercises every other day. Rest for at least 60 seconds between sets.
- Perform 2 sets of bodyweight squats (12-15 reps) every day. Rest for at least 60 seconds between sets.
- Females drink 6 cups of water and 3 cups of green tea every day. Males drink 10 cups of water and 3 cups of green tea every day.
- Set aside 6 minutes every day for focused breathing.
- Find 5 minutes every day to spend in the sun.
- If you typically eat red meat every day, aim to cut out red meat for an entire day at least 3x this week.
- Make sure you are eating at least two servings of fruit and two servings of vegetables every day.

Week 7

- Eat oatmeal for breakfast every day.
- Walk briskly for 30 minutes every day.
- Perform 3 sets (12-16 reps) of bicep curls. Perform 3 sets of overhead presses (12-16 reps). Perform 3 sets (10-16 reps) of tricep kickbacks or overhead tricep extensions. Perform these exercises every other day. Rest for at least 60 seconds between sets.
- Perform 2 sets of bodyweight squats (12-15 reps) every day. Rest for at least 60 seconds between sets.
- Females drink 6 cups of water and 3 cups of green tea every day. Males drink 10 cups of water and 3 cups of green tea every day.
- Set aside 6 minutes every day for focused breathing.
- Find 5 minutes every day to spend in the sun.
- If you typically eat red meat every day, aim to cut out red meat for an entire day at least 4x this week.
- Make sure you are eating at least two servings of fruit and three servings of vegetables every day.

Week 8

- Eat oatmeal for breakfast every day.
- Walk briskly for 30 minutes every day.
- Perform 3 sets (12-16 reps) of bicep curls. Perform 3 sets of overhead presses (12-16 reps). Perform 3 sets (10-16 reps) of tricep kickbacks or overhead tricep extensions. Perform these exercises every other day. Rest for at least 60 seconds between sets.
- Perform 2 sets of bodyweight squats (12-15 reps) every day. Rest for at least 60 seconds between sets.
- Females drink 6 cups of water and 3 cups of green tea every day. Males drink 10 cups of water and 3 cups of green tea every day.
- Set aside 7 minutes every day for focused breathing.
- Find 5 minutes every day to spend in the sun.
- If you typically eat red meat every day, aim to cut out red meat for an entire day at least 4x this week.
- Make sure you are eating at least two servings of fruit and three servings of vegetables every day.

Week 9

- Eat oatmeal for breakfast every day.
- Walk briskly for 30 minutes every day.
- Perform 3 sets (12-16 reps) of bicep curls. Perform 3 sets of overhead presses (12-16 reps). Perform 3 sets (10-16 reps) of tricep kickbacks or overhead tricep extensions. Perform these exercises every other day. Rest for at least 60 seconds between sets.
- Perform 2 sets of bodyweight squats (12-15 reps) every day. Rest for at least 60 seconds between sets.
- Females drink 6 cups of water and 3 cups of green tea every day. Males drink 10 cups of water and 3 cups of green tea every day.
- Set aside 7 minutes every day for focused breathing.
- Find 5 minutes every day to spend in the sun.
- If you typically eat red meat every day, aim to cut out red meat for an entire day at least 5x this week.
- Make sure you are eating at least three servings of fruit and three servings of vegetables every day.

Week 10

- Eat oatmeal for breakfast every day.
- Walk briskly for 30 minutes every day.
- Perform 3 sets (12-16 reps) of bicep curls. Perform 3 sets of overhead presses (12-16 reps). Perform 3 sets (10-16 reps) of tricep kickbacks or overhead tricep extensions. Perform these exercises every other day. Rest for at least 60 seconds between sets.
- Perform 3 sets of bodyweight squats (12-15 reps) every day. Rest for at least 60 seconds between sets.
- Females drink 6 cups of water and 3 cups of green tea every day. Males drink 10 cups of water and 3 cups of green tea every day.
- Set aside 7 minutes every day for focused breathing.
- Find 5 minutes every day to spend in the sun.
- If you typically eat red meat every day, aim to cut out red meat for an entire day at least 5x this week.
- Make sure you are eating at least three servings of fruit and three servings of vegetables every day.

Week 11

- Eat oatmeal for breakfast every day.
- Walk briskly for 30 minutes every day.
- Perform 3 sets (12-16 reps) of bicep curls. Perform 3 sets of overhead presses (12-16 reps). Perform 3 sets (10-16 reps) of tricep kickbacks or overhead tricep extensions. Perform these exercises every other day. Rest for at least 60 seconds between sets.
- Perform 3 sets of bodyweight squats (12-15 reps) every day. Rest for at least 60 seconds between sets.
- Females drink 6 cups of water and 3 cups of green tea every day. Males drink 10 cups of water and 3 cups of green tea every day.
- Set aside 7 minutes every day for focused breathing.
- Find 5 minutes every day to spend in the sun.
- If you typically eat red meat every day, aim to cut out red meat for an entire day at least 5x this week.
- Make sure you are eating at least three servings of fruit and four servings of vegetables every day.

Week 12

- Eat oatmeal for breakfast every day.
- Walk briskly for 30 minutes every day. 3x during your walk, jog or sprint for 30 seconds (ex. walk for 10 minutes, jog or sprint for 30 seconds, walk another 10, jog or sprint for 30 seconds, walk last ten, finish with 30 second jog or sprint).
- Perform 3 sets (12-16 reps) of bicep curls. Perform 3 sets of overhead presses (12-16 reps). Perform 3 sets (12-16 reps) of tricep kickbacks or overhead tricep extensions. Perform these exercises every other day. Rest for at least 60 seconds between sets.
- Perform 3 sets of bodyweight squats (12-15 reps) every day. Rest for at least 60 seconds between sets.
- Females drink 6 cups of water and 3 cups of green tea every day. Males drink 10 cups of water and 3 cups of green tea every day.
- Set aside 7 minutes every day for focused breathing.
- Find 5 minutes every day to spend in the sun.
- If you typically eat red meat every day, aim to cut out red meat for an entire day at least 5x this week.
- Make sure you are eating at least three servings of fruit and four servings of vegetables every day.

Week 13

- Eat oatmeal for breakfast every day.
- Walk briskly for 30 minutes every day. 3x during your walk, jog or sprint for 30 seconds.
- Perform 3 sets (12-16 reps) of bicep curls. Perform 3 sets of overhead presses (12-16 reps). Perform 3 sets (12-16 reps) of tricep kickbacks or overhead extensions. Perform these exercises every other day. Rest for at least 60 seconds between sets.
- Perform 2 sets of bodyweight squats (12-15 reps) every day. Rest for at least 60 seconds between sets. Perform 1 set of dumbbell squats (holding hand weights with your arms straight, at your sides) (12-15 reps). Start with light weights. Increase the amount of weight you use once this exercise becomes easy for you. Perform these exercises every day.
- Females drink 6 cups of water and 3 cups of green tea every day. Males drink 10 cups of water and 3 cups of green tea every day.
- Set aside 7 minutes every day for focused breathing.
- Find 5 minutes every day to spend in the sun.
- If you typically eat red meat every day, aim to cut out red meat for an entire day at least 5x this week.
- Make sure you are eating at least three servings of fruit and four servings of vegetables every day.

Week 14

- Eat oatmeal for breakfast every day.
- Walk briskly for 30 minutes every day. 3x during your walk, jog or sprint for 30 seconds.
- Perform 3 sets (12-16 reps) of bicep curls. Perform 3 sets of overhead presses (12-16 reps). Perform 3 sets (12-16 reps) of tricep kickbacks or overhead extensions. Perform these exercises every other day. Rest for at least 60 seconds between sets.
- Perform 2 sets of bodyweight squats (12-15 reps) and 1 set of dumbbell squats (12-15 reps) every day. Rest for at least 60 seconds between sets.
- Females drink 6 cups of water and 3 cups of green tea every day. Males drink 10 cups of water and 3 cups of green tea every day.
- Set aside 7 minutes every day for focused breathing.
- Find 5 minutes every day to spend in the sun.
- If you typically eat red meat every day, aim to cut out red meat for an entire day at least 5x this week.
- Make sure you are eating at least three servings of fruit and four servings of vegetables every day.

Week 15

- Eat oatmeal for breakfast every day.
- Walk briskly for 30 minutes every day. 3x during your walk, jog or sprint for 45 seconds.
- Perform 3 sets (12-16 reps) of bicep curls. Perform 3 sets of overhead presses (12-16 reps). Perform 3 sets (12-16 reps) of tricep kickbacks or overhead extensions. Perform these exercises every other day. Rest for at least 60 seconds between sets.
- Perform 3 sets of bodyweight squats (12-15 reps) and 1 set of dumbbell squats (12-15 reps) every day. Rest for at least 60 seconds between sets.
- Females drink 6 cups of water and 3 cups of green tea every day. Males drink 10 cups of water and 3 cups of green tea every day.
- Set aside 7 minutes every day for focused breathing.
- Find 5 minutes every day to spend in the sun.
- If you typically eat red meat every day, aim to cut out red meat for an entire day at least 5x this week.
- Make sure you are eating at least three servings of fruit and four servings of vegetables every day.

Week 16

- Eat oatmeal for breakfast every day.
- Walk briskly for 30 minutes every day. 3x during your walk, jog or sprint for 45 seconds.
- Perform 3 sets (12-16 reps) of bicep curls. Perform 3 sets of overhead presses (12-16 reps). Perform 3 sets (12-16 reps) of tricep kickbacks or overhead extensions. Perform these exercises every other day. Rest for at least 60 seconds between sets.
- Perform 3 sets of bodyweight squats (12-15 reps) and 1 set of dumbbell squats (12-15 reps) every day. Rest for at least 60 seconds between sets.
- Females drink 6 cups of water and 3 cups of green tea every day. Males drink 10 cups of water and 3 cups of green tea every day.
- Set aside 7 minutes every day for focused breathing.
- Find 5 minutes every day to spend in the sun.
- If you typically eat red meat every day, aim to cut out red meat for an entire day at least 5x this week.
- Make sure you are eating at least three servings of fruit and four servings of vegetables every day.

Week 17

- Eat oatmeal for breakfast every day.
- Walk briskly for 30 minutes every day. 3x during your walk, jog or sprint for 45 seconds.
- Perform 3 sets (12-16 reps) of bicep curls. Perform 3 sets of overhead presses (12-16 reps). Perform 3 sets (12-16 reps) of tricep kickbacks or overhead extensions. Perform these exercises every other day. Rest for at least 60 seconds between sets.
- Perform 3 sets of bodyweight squats (12-15 reps) and 2 sets of dumbbell squats (12-15 reps) every day. Rest for at least 60 seconds between sets.
- Females drink 6 cups of water and 3 cups of green tea every day. Males drink 10 cups of water and 3 cups of green tea every day.
- Set aside 7 minutes every day for focused breathing.
- Find 5 minutes every day to spend in the sun.
- If you typically eat red meat every day, aim to cut out red meat for an entire day at least 5x this week.
- Make sure you are eating at least three servings of fruit and four servings of vegetables every day.

Week 18

- Eat oatmeal for breakfast every day.
- Walk briskly for 30 minutes every day. 3x during your walk, jog or sprint for 60 seconds.
- Perform 3 sets (12-16 reps) of bicep curls. Perform 3 sets of overhead presses (12-16 reps). Perform 3 sets (12-16 reps) of tricep kickbacks or overhead extensions. Perform these exercises every other day. Rest for at least 60 seconds between sets.
- Perform 3 sets of bodyweight squats (12-15 reps) and 2 sets of dumbbell squats (12-15 reps) every day. Rest for at least 60 seconds between sets.
- Females drink 6 cups of water and 3 cups of green tea every day. Males drink 10 cups of water and 3 cups of green tea every day.
- Set aside 7 minutes every day for focused breathing.
- Find 5 minutes every day to spend in the sun.
- If you typically eat red meat every day, aim to cut out red meat for an entire day at least 5x this week.
- Make sure you are eating at least three servings of fruit and four servings of vegetables every day.

Week 19

- Eat oatmeal for breakfast every day.
- Walk briskly for 30 minutes every day. 3x during your walk, jog or sprint for 60 seconds.
- Perform 3 sets (12-16 reps) of bicep curls. Perform 3 sets of overhead presses (12-16 reps). Perform 3 sets (12-16 reps) of tricep kickbacks or overhead extensions. Perform these exercises every other day. Rest for at least 60 seconds between sets.
- Perform 3 sets of bodyweight squats (12-15 reps) and 2 sets of dumbbell squats (12-15 reps) every day. Rest for at least 60 seconds between sets.
- Females drink 6 cups of water and 3 cups of green tea every day. Males drink 10 cups of water and 3 cups of green tea every day.
- Set aside 7 minutes every day for focused breathing.
- Find 5 minutes every day to spend in the sun.
- If you typically eat red meat every day, aim to cut out red meat for an entire day at least 5x this week.
- Make sure you are eating at least three servings of fruit and four servings of vegetables every day.

Week 20

- Eat oatmeal for breakfast every day.
- Walk briskly for 30 minutes every day. 3x during your walk, jog or sprint for 60 seconds.
- Perform 3 sets (12-16 reps) of bicep curls. Perform 3 sets of overhead presses (12-16 reps). Perform 3 sets (12-16 reps) of tricep kickbacks or overhead extensions. Perform these exercises every other day. Rest for at least 60 seconds between sets.
- Perform 3 sets of bodyweight squats (12-15 reps) and 3 sets of dumbbell squats (12-15 reps) every day. Rest for at least 60 seconds between sets.
- Females drink 6 cups of water and 3 cups of green tea every day. Males drink 10 cups of water and 3 cups of green tea every day.
- Set aside 7 minutes every day for focused breathing.
- Find 5 minutes every day to spend in the sun.
- If you typically eat red meat every day, aim to cut out red meat for an entire day at least 5x this week.
- Make sure you are eating at least three servings of fruit and four servings of vegetables every day.

From now on: continue with Week 20, adjusting the amount of weight, sets, or repetitions as needed, increasing your bouts of jogging; or create your own program based upon your abilities, likes, and dislikes.

Bibliography

Giovannucci E, Liu Y, Hollis BW, Rimm EB. 25-hydroxyvitamin D and risk of myocardial infarction in men: a prospective study. Arch Intern Med. 2008; 168:1174-80.

Kaplan, N.M & Victor, R.G. (2010). Kaplan's Clinical Hypertension (10th ed.). Baltimore, MD.: Wolters Kluwer/ Lippincott Williams & Wilkins

Kuriyama S, Shimazu T, Ohmori K, et al. Green Tea Consumption and Mortality Due to Cardiovascular Disease, Cancer, and All Causes in Japan: The Ohsaki Study. JAMA. 2006;296(10):1255-1265. doi:10.1001/jama.296.10.1255.

Pan, A., Sun, Q., Bernstein, A. M., Schulze, M. B., Manson, J. E., Stampfer, M. J., ... Hu, F. B. (2012). Red Meat Consumption and Mortality: Results from Two Prospective Cohort Studies. Archives of Internal Medicine, 172(7), 555–563. http://doi.org/10.1001/archinternmed.2011.2287

Pereira MA, O'Reilly E, Augustsson K, et al. Dietary Fiber and Risk of Coronary Heart Disease: A Pooled Analysis of Cohort Studies. Arch Intern Med. 2004;164(4):370-376. doi: 10.1001/archinte.164.4.370.